ANDYN N. DANG

FIT FOR LIFE: 5 SIMPLE STEPS TO ESTABLISH A DAILY WORKOUT HABIT

20 Minutes Daily Workout To Lose Weight, Enhance Muscle Strength, Endurance, Flexibility & Boost Energy

First published by GrwMindSetPress 2024

Copyright © 2024 by Andyn N. Dang

All rights reserved. No part of this publication may be reproduced, stored or transmitted in any form or by any means, electronic, mechanical, photocopying, recording, scanning, or otherwise without written permission from the publisher. It is illegal to copy this book, post it to a website, or distribute it by any other means without permission.

Andyn N. Dang asserts the moral right to be identified as the author of this work.

Andyn N. Dang has no responsibility for the persistence or accuracy of URLs for external or third-party Internet Websites referred to in this publication and does not guarantee that any content on such Websites is, or will remain, accurate or appropriate.

Designations used by companies to distinguish their products are often claimed as trademarks. All brand names and product names used in this book and on its cover are trade names, service marks, trademarks and registered trademarks of their respective owners. The publishers and the book are not associated with any product or vendor mentioned in this book. None of the companies referenced within the book have endorsed the book.

Third edition

*This book was professionally typeset on Reedsy.
Find out more at reedsy.com*

Contents

Introduction	1
Chapter I	3
1. The Science of Habit Formation	3
2. Navigating the Challenges of Habit Formation	7
Chapter II	10
1. Crafting Your Unique Exercise Routine: A Personalized Approach to Fitness	10
2. Finding Joy in Movement	12
3. Embracing Consistency	13
4. Samples YouTube Workout Routine:	15
Chapter III	17
1. Understanding the Why	17
2. Setting SMART Goals [3]	18
3. Categorizing Fitness Goals	19
4. Monitoring and Adjusting	19
Chapter IV	23
1: The Art of Starting Small	23
2: Overcoming Psychological Barriers	24
3: Progression and Scaling Up	25
4: Cultivating Momentum	25
5: Navigating Setbacks	26
Chapter V	28
1. The Catalyst of Accountability:	28
2. Shared Goals, Shared Triumphs:	29
3. Virtual Accountability:	29

4. Professional Guidance and Support:	30
5. The Power of Encouragement:	30
Conclusion	32

Introduction

Welcome to "Fit for Life." In the following pages, we embark on a transformative exploration of two pillars that lay the foundation for a healthier, more fulfilling existence: the importance and benefits of daily exercise and the cultivation of a positive mindset to achieve sustainable habits. In understanding the profound impact of daily physical activity on our well-being, we unravel the intricacies of how exercise serves as a catalyst for enhanced physical health, mental clarity, and emotional resilience. Simultaneously, we delve into the psychology of habits, exploring how fostering a positive mindset creates a harmonious environment for achievable and lasting habits. This book is more than a guide; it's an invitation to discover the synergistic relationship between the movement of our bodies and the thoughts in our minds, empowering you to embark on a journey of holistic wellness and self-discovery. Let's elevate our lives together, one step and positive habit at a time.

Our first chapter, "Understanding the Psychology of Habits," delves into the Science of Habit Formation. Together, we unravel the neural intricacies that shape our behaviors, providing you with a foundational understanding of the forces that drive our daily actions. As we embark on this exploration, we equip you with the tools to overcome common challenges, laying the groundwork for transformative change.

Chapter II, "Creating a Consistent Workout Routine," invites you to establish an exercise routine that resonates with your unique style. We explore the art of setting a regular schedule for daily workouts, infusing intention into each session. Additionally, we guide you in establishing a dedicated workout space—a personal sanctuary that elevates your commitment to holistic well-being.

In Chapter III, "Setting Clear Fitness Goals," we shift our focus to the power of purpose. Specific, measurable, and realistic goals become the focal point of your daily exercise, while short-term and long-term objectives provide a compass for your wellness journey. With clarity in your aspirations, you're poised to achieve meaningful and sustainable results.

As we progress to Chapter IV, "Starting Small and Building Momentum," the journey becomes a gradual ascent. We explore the beauty of a gentle introduction to exercise and strategies for increasing intensity, ensuring that each step is not only manageable but also a building block for sustained progress.

In Chapter V, "Leveraging Accountability and Support," we recognize the strength of partnership. Discover the benefits of a workout buddy—a companion on your fitness journey—and explore techniques for self-accountability that empower you to stay committed, even in the face of challenges.

"Fit for Life" is more than a guide; it's an invitation to re-imagine your relationship with health and fitness. Each chapter unfolds a new layer of possibility, encouraging you to embrace a mindful approach to movement and well-being. As you embark on this journey, envision "Fit for Life" as your companion—a source of inspiration, knowledge, and empowerment on your path to a healthier, more balanced life. Let's explore the transformative synergy of mind and body as we embrace mindful movement together. Welcome to a journey where each step is a mindful stride toward wellness.

Chapter I

Understanding the Psychology of Habits

"Motivation is what gets you started. Habit is what keeps you going." – Jim Ryun

1. The Science of Habit Formation

In the vast expanse of our brains, a symphony of neurons orchestrates the intricate dance of habit formation. Understanding this neural ballet is paramount as we unravel the science behind the habits that shape our lives.

The Habit Loop: Cue, Routine, Reward[1]

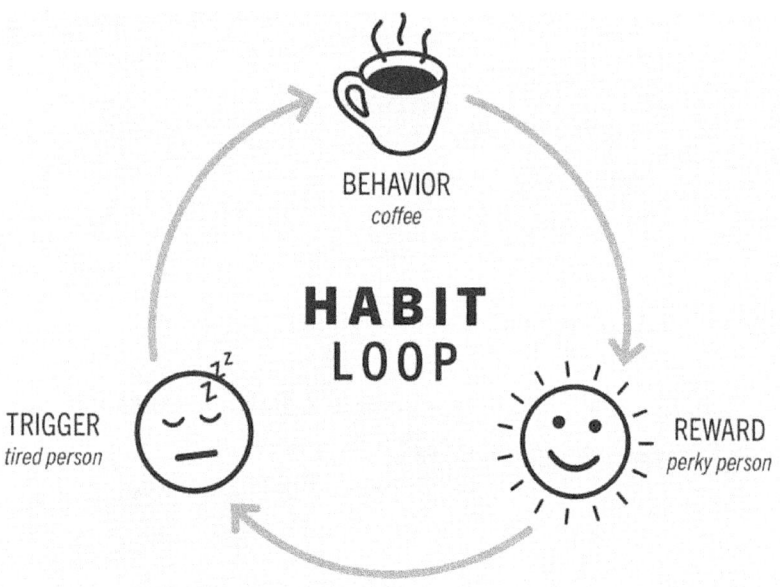

At the core of habit formation lies the habit loop—a neurological sequence consisting of three key components:

- **The Cue:** A catalyst that triggers the habit loop.
- **The Routine:** This is the behavior, the action taken in response to the cue.
- **The Reward:** The most critical component. It is the benefit derived from the behavior. It reinforces the loop and ensures its repetition.

This loop becomes etched into the neural pathways, solidifying the habit through a process known as synaptic plasticity.

CHAPTER I

Cue: The Triggering Signal

This is the WHY. Understanding your cues is paramount to altering or establishing habits. Cues initiate the habit loop. The two most common cues are *fear & desire*.

One example is how we established our habit of brushing our teeth every night and every morning without thinking about it. The primary cues are the *fear* of toothache and bad breath—the *desire* for healthy teeth. I apply a similar *fear* trigger to forge my daily workout into a habit to avoid fatigue and sluggishness. I apply the same *desire* for good health and maintain my daily energy to stay productive.

Another example is considering that our body and mind are like our phone's hardware and software. How can we all establish the habit of charging our phones every night so quickly? The cue is we *fear* our phones will run out of battery during the day, and our *desire* to keep our phones full battery so they can function optimally throughout the day. We are all taking good care of our precious phones since we are so dependent on them in today's world. Our bodies & minds are 100 times more important than our phones. If we apply the same *fear* that our bodies & minds will also run out of energy during the day and the same *desire* for our bodies & minds to run optimally and productively throughout the day, we are all can kick-start a daily workout habit as a snap of a finger without 2nd though, shouldn't we?

Routine: The Neural Choreography

Once the cue is received, the routine takes center stage. This is the HOW and WHAT. It is the habitual behavior or action prompted by the cue. As you repeatedly engage in this routine, the neural pathways associated with it become more defined and efficient, reducing the cognitive load required for execution. The brain, in its remarkable efficiency, seeks to conserve energy by automating these routines.

Establishing a *routine* that resonates with your preferences and brings you joy is very important. It helps you carry out effortlessly without thinking about it every time. I recommend building and optimizing your daily exercise routine by searching YouTube videos for Yoga, Tai Chi, Qigong, Cardio exercise, and breathing techniques. Look for five to six simple moves that resonate with you.my recommendation is to search for two movements that target the neck, shoulder, and upper body: one for abs, one for cardio, one for lower body strength, and the last one for breathing technique. Start with three minutes for each movement. The key is to focus your energy on the target body part that each movement is intended for throughout the workout; that way, you can feel the effectiveness and have measurable satisfaction results. The best way is to start with small, short 15–20 minutes daily to reinforce consistency over intensity and gradually increase when the habit has been established. The key is joy and satisfaction to maintain consistency.

Reward: The Neurochemical Payoff

The reward serves as the grand finale. The joy, satisfaction, energetic feeling, and refreshment that result after each workout release a surge of neurochemicals to reinforce the habit loop. Dopamine, the neurotransmitter associated with pleasure and reward, plays a pivotal role. It creates a sense of satisfaction and reinforces the brain's association between the cue and the routine, making the habit loop more likely to be re-activated.

The Role of Basal Ganglia[2]: The Habitual Maestro

Deep within the brain, the basal ganglia emerges as the conductor of this neurological symphony. Responsible for procedural learning and motor control, this cluster of nuclei becomes the epicenter for habit formation. As habits become ingrained, the basal ganglia takes charge, allowing us to execute routines with minimal conscious effort.

CHAPTER I

Neuroplasticity [2]: Rewiring the Brain's Blueprint
The brain's ability to adapt and reorganize itself is known as neuroplasticity. As habits form, the neural connections associated with them strengthen, creating well-trodden paths that facilitate the habit loop. Understanding neuroplasticity empowers us to intentionally shape our neural landscape, fostering the growth of positive habits while pruning the pathways of detrimental ones.

In the subsequent chapters, we will explore strategies to leverage this neurological understanding for effective habit formation. From manipulating cues to optimizing rewards, each element of the habit loop becomes a tool for sculpting the habits that lead to personal and professional excellence. As we continue this exploration, remember that the science of habit formation is not merely an academic pursuit but a practical guide to transforming your life, one neural pathway at a time.

2.Navigating the Challenges of Habit Formation

As you embark on the transformative journey of habit formation, several common challenges may arise. To guide you through these hurdles, let's focus on five key obstacles and effective strategies for overcoming them:

Ambitious Goal Setting: Start Small, Specific, Aim Big

- **Challenge:** Setting overly ambitious goals can lead to frustration and burnout.
- **Strategy:** Begin with micro-habits—tiny, specific, and achievable actions that lay the foundation for larger changes. Gradually scale up as these small steps become ingrained in your routine.

- **Example:** Instead of "exercise more," specify "walk for 30 minutes every morning."

Inconsistent Routine: Anchor Habits to Existing Activities

- **Challenge:** Inconsistency in routine can hinder habit formation.
- **Strategy:** Align your new habits with existing routines. Use established daily activities as cues to seamlessly integrate your habits into your day, ensuring a consistent and sustainable approach.
- **Example**: If you want to develop a reading habit, link it to your morning coffee.

Lack of Motivation: Connect to Intrinsic Motivations

- **Challenge:** Sustaining motivation over time can be challenging.
- **Strategy**: Identify the intrinsic motivations behind your habits. Visualize the positive outcomes and remind yourself why these habits matter. Cultivating intrinsic motivation transforms habits from mere tasks into meaningful components of personal growth.
- **Example:** Instead of focusing your daily exercise solely on external goals like weight loss, shift your perspective to the joy of each movement and its positive impact on your overall body, health, and well-being.

Progress Tracking: Celebrate Small Wins

- **Challenge:** Lack of progress tracking may lead to a lack of accountability.
- **Strategy:** Implement a tracking system, whether it's a habit-tracking app, journal, or calendar. Celebrate each small victory along the way. This will provide accountability and serve as a

tangible record of your journey, showcasing the strides you've made.
- **Example:** Use activity tracking apps to track your movements or just a simple checkoff on a physical calendar at your workout space. This will give you a sense of self-reward for your accomplishment.

Adaptability: Thriving in Change

- **Challenge:** Life's unpredictability can disrupt established routines.
- **Strategy:** Cultivate adaptability by developing alternative strategies for maintaining habits during unexpected challenges. An adaptable approach ensures continued progress in the face of change.
- **Example:** If you can't find 30 minutes for your workout due to unforeseen work commitments or family emergencies, break your workout into shorter, more manageable sessions. Aim for three 10-minute sessions throughout the day to ensure you still get some exercise without feeling overwhelmed.

Addressing the above five common challenges will better equip you to navigate the intricacies of habit formation. Remember, the journey is as much about resilience and adaptability as it is about discipline. As you overcome these obstacles, you'll find yourself on a path of sustainable personal growth and positive change.

Chapter II

Creating a Consistent Workout Routine

"Success isn't always about greatness. It's about consistency. Consistent hard work leads to success. Greatness will come."
– Dwayne "The Rock" Johnson

1. Crafting Your Unique Exercise Routine: A Personalized Approach to Fitness

Embarking on a fitness journey is a profoundly personal endeavor. The quest for a sustainable and enjoyable exercise routine necessitates a tailored approach—one that aligns with your preferences, lifestyle, and individual needs. In this chapter, we'll explore the art of formulating a bespoke exercise routine that not only enhances your physical well-being but also harmoniously aligns with your unique style.

Chapter II

Understanding Your Preferences

Self-Reflection:

Take a moment to reflect on your past experiences with exercise. What activities bring you joy? Are you drawn to the energy of group classes, the solitude of nature walks, or the intensity of weight training? Understanding your preferences lays the foundation for a routine you'll be excited to embrace.

Setting Realistic Goals:

Define your fitness goals, keeping them realistic and achievable. Whether it's improving cardiovascular health, building strength, or simply incorporating more movement into your day, clear goals will guide the structure of your routine.

Designing Your Routine

- **Variety for Engagement:**

Inject variety into your routine to prevent monotony. Blend cardiovascular exercises, strength training, flexibility work, and activities you genuinely enjoy. A mix of elements keeps your routine engaging and caters to different aspects of fitness.

- **Scheduling:**

Consider your daily schedule and energy levels. Are you a morning person eager to start the day with a workout, or do you find solace in an evening routine? Tailor your exercise schedule to sync with your natural rhythms for enhanced consistency.

- **Flexibility and Adaptability:**

Life is dynamic, and so should be your exercise routine. Craft a flexible plan that accommodates unexpected changes in your schedule or preferences. Embrace adaptability as a key component of a sustainable routine.

- **Establishing a dedicated Workout Space:**

Creating a dedicated workout space is akin to crafting a sanctuary for physical well-being. This personalized haven, whether it's a corner in your living room or a converted spare room, serves as a tangible manifestation of your commitment to health. The atmosphere is intentionally curated with motivational elements—perhaps a wall adorned with fitness quotes, a mirror reflecting determination, or the subtle hum of uplifting music. In this sacred space, the outside world fades, allowing the focus to shift inward. The mere act of stepping into this realm signals a transition from the demands of daily life to a dedicated time for self-improvement. The workout space becomes a canvas for movement, where sweat transforms into accomplishment, and each routine becomes a brushstroke in the masterpiece of your fitness journey. It's not just a physical space; it's a mental refuge—a place where intentions align with actions and the pursuit of well-being unfolds with purpose and dedication.

2.Finding Joy in Movement

Joyful Activities:
Identify activities that bring you genuine joy. Whether it's dancing, hiking, cycling, or practicing yoga, incorporating activities you love transforms exercise from a chore into a source of pleasure.

Social or Solo:
Consider your social preferences. Some thrive in the camaraderie of group classes, while others find solace in solo pursuits. Tailor your routine to your social inclinations to ensure a supportive and enjoyable fitness environment.

Listening to Your Body

- **Intuitive Exercise:**

Cultivate a mindful approach to exercise by listening to your body. Pay close attention to how different activities make you feel physically and emotionally. Focus your the energy flow to the body part where your movement is intended for. Adjust your routine based on your body's cues and needs.

- **Rest and Recovery:**

Recognize the importance of rest and recovery in your routine. Integrate rest days and prioritize quality sleep to support your body's healing and adaptation process.

3.Embracing Consistency

Establishing Habits:
Aligning your routine with your daily rituals can transform it into a habit. Whether it's a morning jog, a lunchtime stretch, or an evening workout, consistency fosters the integration of exercise into your lifestyle.
The time it takes to establish a habit can vary widely from person to person, and there isn't a universally agreed-upon duration. The

idea that it takes 21 days to form a habit is a common belief, but it's not backed by robust scientific evidence. In reality, the time required to establish a habit can range from several weeks to several months, depending on each individual.

Research published in the European Journal of Social Psychology in 2009 suggested that, on average, it takes about 66 days for a new behavior to become automatic or a habit. However, this was an average, and individual variations were considerable, ranging from 18 to 254 days.

Several factors can influence the time it takes to establish a habit:

- **Behavior Complexity:** Simple behaviors may become habits more quickly than complex ones.
- **Frequency:** The more frequently a behavior is repeated, the more likely it becomes a habit.
- **Consistency:** Regular and consistent practice reinforces habit formation.
- **Personal Motivation:** Intrinsic motivation and a strong personal desire to form a habit can accelerate the process.
- **Behavioral Cues**: Habits can form more effectively if they are linked to specific cues or triggers in your environment or daily routine.
- **Previous Habit-Forming Experience:** Individuals who have successfully formed habits in the past may find it easier to establish new ones.

It's essential to be patient and realistic when trying to establish a habit. Celebrate small victories along the way, and understand that setbacks are a normal part of the process. Additionally, the concept of habit formation is ongoing, and habits can be refined or adjusted over time

CHAPTER II

to better suit your goals and lifestyle.

Celebrating Progress:
Celebrate the small victories along your fitness journey. Progress may not always be linear, but acknowledging and appreciating your achievements reinforces your commitment to your unique exercise routine.

In conclusion, your exercise routine is an expression of self-care and a reflection of your unique style. By understanding your preferences, setting realistic goals, and infusing joy into your movement, you create a sustainable and fulfilling approach to fitness—one that stands the test of time and aligns seamlessly with the individual that you are.

4.Samples YouTube Workout Routine:

20 min Cardio Full Body Workout Routine:
https://www.youtube.com/watch?v=FeR-4_Opt-g
20 Minute Full Body Cardio HIIT Workout:
https://www.youtube.com/watch?v=M0uO8X3_tEA
30 min Zumba Latin dance:
https://www.youtube.com/watch?v=mZeFvX3ALKY
30 min Zumba Latin dance Workout for beginners:
https://youtu.be/e5rW7qjd3BY?si=IPjcQspoqNXiJRSR
15 Minutes Dance Party Workout - Full Body:
https://youtu.be/1vRto-2MMZo?si=CLkJt3qUAV38eXS9
20 min Fat Burning Workout for Total Beginners:
https://youtu.be/IT94xC35u6k?si=MkbVtMWrrEt5XYov
15 min daily full body Stretching routine:
https://youtu.be/g_tea8ZNk5A?si=DHqcpT-7mzh4CI6M
15 Min. Pilates Workout - Slow Full Body Toning:
https://www.youtube.com/watch?v=f9UbVRqd9YY

20 Min. Express Pilates Workout ‖ Everyday Pilates For Energy
https://www.youtube.com/watch?v=ezke0GlKeM4
Morning Yoga Workout Better Than The Gym | Strength & Stretch
https://www.youtube.com/watch?v=oX6I6vs1EFs

Chapter III

Clarity in Motion: Setting Clear Fitness Goals

"Every day is another chance to get stronger, to eat better, to live healthier, and to be the best version of you." – Unknown

Embarking on a fitness journey without clear goals is akin to navigating uncharted waters without a compass. In this chapter, we delve into the profound importance of setting explicit fitness goals—ones that act as beacons, guiding your efforts, shaping your routines, and propelling you toward lasting change.

1. Understanding the Why

Reflecting on Intentions:
Unveil the deeper motivations behind your fitness journey. Whether you're achieving a healthier lifestyle, building strength, or boosting confidence, understanding the core reasons fuels a sense of purpose that anchors your goals.

Aligning with Values:

Connect your fitness goals with your core values. When your pursuits align with what truly matters to you, the journey becomes more meaningful and sustainable.

2. Setting SMART Goals [3]

Specificity:

Craft goals with precision. Instead of a vague aim like "lose weight," articulate specific targets like "run a 5K in under 30 minutes."

Measurability:

Establish concrete metrics to track progress. Whether it's tracking miles, recording weights, or monitoring workout frequency, measurable goals offer clarity and accountability. For example, "complete 20 push-ups every morning."

Achievability:

Ensure your goals are realistic and attainable. Striking a balance between challenge and achievability prevents discouragement and fosters a sense of accomplishment.

Relevance:

Assess the relevance of your goals to your overarching fitness journey. Each goal should contribute to the larger narrative of your well-being.

Time-Bound:

Infuse your goals with a temporal dimension. Setting deadlines creates a sense of urgency and aids in structuring your fitness road-map.

3. Categorizing Fitness Goals

Comprehensive Wellness:
Your goals should encompass various dimensions of wellness, including cardiovascular health, strength training, flexibility, and mental well-being. A holistic approach ensures a balanced and sustainable fitness routine.

Short-Term vs. Long-Term:
Distinguish between short-term achievements and long-term aspirations. Short-term goals provide stepping stones, while long-term visions shape the overarching trajectory of your fitness journey.

4. Monitoring and Adjusting

Regular Assessment:
Periodically evaluate your progress. Adjust goals based on achievements, setbacks, and evolving priorities to keep your fitness journey dynamic and responsive.

Celebrating Milestones:
Celebrate each milestone, regardless of size. Acknowledging achievements reinforces positive behavior and serves as motivation for continued progress.

In conclusion, setting clear fitness goals is the compass that guides your journey toward optimal well-being. By understanding your motivations, employing SMART criteria, and embracing a comprehensive approach, your goals become not just targets but integral components of a transformative fitness narrative. As you navigate this chapter, consider it a road-map that leads to a healthier, more vital, and more vibrant version of yourself.

MAKE A DIFFERENCE WITH YOUR REVIEW

"A single act of kindness throws out roots in all directions, and the roots spring up and make new trees." – Amelia Earhart

Fit for Life: 5 Simple Steps to Establish a Daily Workout Habit is more than just a guide—it's a beacon of hope and motivation for anyone ready to make a lasting change in their life. And now, you have the power to make a difference.

Your experience with this book can inspire others. By leaving a review, you're not just sharing your thoughts—you're shining a light for someone else who's ready to embark on their fitness journey. Your words could be the encouragement they need to take that first step toward a healthier life.

I humbly ask for your help. Be the motivation that someone else needs to start their fitness journey. Most people decide to read a book based on the reviews, and your review could be the push they need to begin their transformation.

By taking just 1 minute to leave a review, you're contributing to a ripple effect of positive change. Your review could help…

…one more person finds the motivation to start working out.

…one more person achieves their fitness goals.

…one more person feels healthier and happier.

To make a difference, all you need to do is…

Kindly Leave a Review:

For ebook: https://www.amazon.com/review/review-your-purchases/?asin=B0CXMV8ZDV

OR Scan the QR code:

CHAPTER III

If helping others resonates with you, you're my kind of person. Welcome to the community of those who believe in the power of positive change.

I'm thrilled that **Fit for Life** can be a part of your journey. I hope it has inspired and guided you as much as I believe it can. And I'm even more excited about the incredible impact your review could have on someone else's life. Thank you for being a part of this journey and for helping others along the way.

For Paperback: https://www.amazon.com/review/review-your-purchases/?asin=B0CXMPC3HS

OR simply scan the QR code below to leave your review:

FIT FOR LIFE: 5 SIMPLE STEPS TO ESTABLISH A DAILY WORKOUT HABIT

If helping others resonates with you, you're my kind of person. Welcome to the community of those who believe in the power of positive change.

I'm thrilled that **Fit for Life** can be a part of your journey. I hope it has inspired and guided you as much as I believe it can. And I'm even more excited about the incredible impact your review could have on someone else's life. Thank you for being a part of this journey and for helping others along the way.

Chapter IV

Starting Small and Building Momentum

"Strive for progress, not perfection." – Unknown

Welcome to a chapter dedicated to beginning your fitness journey with modest steps and gradually building a powerful momentum that will propel you toward a consistent and rewarding daily exercise habit. In this chapter, we'll explore the psychology of starting small, understand the impact of incremental progress, and provide practical examples to guide you through the process.

1: The Art of Starting Small

Micro-Habits:

Imagine starting your fitness journey with micro-habits, tiny yet impactful actions that pave the way for more significant changes. For instance, commit to doing just five minutes of stretching every morning or taking a short walk after lunch. These micro-habits are the seeds of your daily exercise routine.

Consistency Over Intensity:
Prioritize consistency in the early stages. Opt for an easy-to-manage daily routine and ensure you stick to it. Whether it's a brief workout video, a short jog, or a set of quick body-weight exercises, the key is to make it a non-negotiable part of your day.

Illustrative Example:

- Micro-Habit: A 5-minute morning stretch routine.
- Consistency: Commit to doing it every day, even on busy mornings.

2: Overcoming Psychological Barriers

Reducing Resistance:
Understand and overcome the resistance often associated with starting something new. More minor actions are less intimidating, making overcoming mental hurdles and initiating your exercise routine easier.

Celebrating Small Wins:
Train your mind to celebrate even the smallest achievements. Completing your micro-habit is a victory worth acknowledging. This positive reinforcement builds a foundation for lasting motivation.

Illustrative Example:

- Psychological Barrier: Feeling overwhelmed by the idea of daily exercise.
- Solution: Break it down into a manageable micro-habit and celebrate each day's completion.

3: Progression and Scaling Up

Gradual Progression:
Explore the concept of gradual progression. Once your micro-habit feels like second nature, consider increasing the duration or intensity. This gradual approach minimizes the risk of burnout.

Successive Goals:
Set achievable goals that align with your growing fitness level. If you started with a 5-minute routine, aim for 10 minutes next. Each goal achieved becomes a stepping stone toward a more active lifestyle.

Illustrative Example:

- Gradual Progression: Increase your 5-minute stretch routine to 7 minutes after two weeks.
- Successive Goals: Aim to reach a 10-minute routine within the next month.

4: Cultivating Momentum

Routine Consistency:
Embed your daily exercise routine into your schedule. Establish a specific time or trigger that signals the start of your workout. The more consistent you are, the more momentum you'll build.

Positive Feedback Loop:
Appreciate the positive feedback loop of consistent exercise. Your motivation grows as you experience the physical and mental benefits,

creating a self-sustaining cycle.

Illustrative Example:

- Consistency: Schedule your 5-minute stretch routine at the same time each morning.
- Feedback Loop: Feel the increased energy and improved mood throughout the day.

5: Navigating Setbacks

Accepting Imperfection:
Embrace the fact that setbacks are a natural part of any journey. Accept imperfection, learn from setbacks, and use them as opportunities for growth.

The Power of Restarting:
Cultivate the power of restarting. If life gets busy or you miss a day, restart without dwelling on guilt. Every restart is a step towards reinforcing your commitment.

Illustrative Example:

- Setback: Missed a workout due to a hectic day.
- Restart: Begin again the next day without self-criticism.

Conclusion: Sustainable Momentum

As we conclude this chapter, envision your daily exercise routine as a dynamic, evolving journey. By starting small and building momentum, you're not just forming a habit but also fostering a wellness lifestyle.

CHAPTER IV

Celebrate the journey, embrace the process, and let the momentum carry you toward a healthier and more active version of yourself.

Chapter V

Leveraging Accountability and Support for Your Daily Exercise Routine

"Fitness is not about being better than someone else. It's about being better than you used to be." – Khloe Kardashian

Power in Partnership:
Getting onto the path to a daily exercise routine is not a solitary endeavor but a shared journey. This chapter explores the transformative influence of accountability and support, providing insights and strategies to fortify your commitment and maintain a consistent exercise habit.

1. The Catalyst of Accountability:

Personal Accountability:
Acknowledge the role of personal accountability. Set clear goals, track progress, and hold yourself responsible for your commitment to daily exercise. The first step in leveraging accountability is recognizing your intrinsic power in shaping your fitness journey.

Accountability Partnerships:

Consider enlisting an accountability partner—a friend, family member, or colleague who shares your fitness aspirations. The mutual commitment creates a shared sense of responsibility, fostering consistency and motivation.

2. Shared Goals, Shared Triumphs:

Defining Shared Objectives:

Establish shared fitness goals with your accountability partner. Whether it's a common target like daily steps or a joint commitment to a fitness class, aligning your objectives enhances motivation and solidarity.

Celebrate Together:

Celebrate achievements collectively. Share triumphs, big or small, and reinforce the positive impact of your shared commitment. Celebrating together strengthens your bond and contributes to a supportive environment.

3. Virtual Accountability:

Online Communities:

Leverage the power of online communities and social media platforms dedicated to fitness. Joining groups or creating your own virtual fitness circle provides a sense of connection, encouragement, and shared accountability.

Tracking Apps and Challenges:
Explore fitness-tracking apps and challenges that allow you to connect with others pursuing similar goals. The gamification of fitness can make the journey more engaging and create a sense of friendly competition.

4. Professional Guidance and Support:

Trainers and Coaches:
Consider seeking guidance from fitness professionals, trainers, or coaches. Their expertise provides structured support, personalized advice, and a professional perspective that can elevate your exercise routine.

Group Fitness Classes:
Engage in group fitness classes, either in-person or virtual. The camaraderie and shared energy in a group setting enhance motivation and accountability, making it more likely for you to adhere to your routine.

5. The Power of Encouragement:

Words of Encouragement:
Exchange words of encouragement with your accountability partner or within your fitness community. Positive affirmations and support create a nurturing environment that propels you forward, especially during challenging times.

Reminders and Check-Ins:
Schedule regular check-ins with your accountability partner. Whether it's a daily text, a weekly call, or a shared calendar, these

CHAPTER V

check-ins serve as gentle reminders and reinforce your commitment. In conclusion, the strength of accountability and support lies in their ability to transform the journey to a daily exercise routine from a solitary pursuit into a collective triumph. By recognizing the power of personal and shared accountability, celebrating achievements together, leveraging virtual communities, seeking professional guidance, and fostering a culture of encouragement, you build a robust foundation for establishing and maintaining a lifelong commitment to daily exercise. As you navigate this chapter, envision your exercise routine not as an individual effort but as a shared endeavor—each step forward is a testament to the strength of partnerships and the collective determination for a healthier, more active lifestyle.

Conclusion

"Take care of your body. It's the only place you have to live."
— Jim Rohn

In our journey together, we've explored the multifaceted world of health and fitness—unveiling the importance and benefits of daily exercise, delving into the power of a positive mindset for achievable habits, unraveling the intricate psychology behind habit formation, and navigating the path to creating a consistent workout routine that aligns with your unique style.

Understanding the science of habit formation equipped us with insights into the neurological symphony that underlies our daily behaviors. At the same time, exploring common challenges provided a roadmap for overcoming obstacles on our way to personal transformation. We ventured into the realm of setting clear fitness goals, emphasizing the specificity, measurability, and realism required for goal setting and the distinction between short-term wins and long-term aspirations.

The chapter on starting small and building momentum encourages a gradual approach to exercise, ensuring that every step is sustainable. Strategies for increasing intensity introduce the concept of progression, highlighting the importance of variety and incremental challenges in our fitness journey.

CONCLUSION

As we approached the conclusion of this book, we recognized the pivotal role of accountability and support. Exploring the benefits of a workout buddy illuminated the strength of partnerships, while techniques for self-accountability provided tools for personal responsibility. Together, we established that the journey to a healthier, more active lifestyle is not solitary but a shared endeavor where encouragement, connection, and commitment intertwine.

In closing, remember that this is not just the end of a book; it's the beginning of a newfound relationship with your well-being. As you venture forth, armed with the knowledge and strategies woven into these pages, envision your future self—committed to daily exercise, guided by clear goals, embracing a positive mindset, and supported by the network of accountability you've cultivated. May each step, each habit formed, and every goal achieved become a testament to your unwavering dedication to a life of vitality and wellness. Here's to your journey, the power within you, and the limitless possibilities that await on the path to a healthier and happier you.

Reference Sources:

[1] *The scoop on the Habit Loop – How to create healthy Habits.* Center for Nutrition Studies. Duncan, O. (2021, March 3).

https://nutritionstudies.org/the-scoop-on-the-habit-loop-how-to-create-healthy-habits/

[2] The brain that changes itself: stories of personal triumph from the frontiers of brain science. *Choice Reviews Online, 45*(10), 45–5559 by Doidge, N. (2008). https://normandoidge.com/?page_id=1259

[3] The ultimate guide to S.M.A.R.T. goals by Leonard, K. & Rob Watts (2022, May 4).

https://www.forbes.com/advisor/business/smart-goals/